DEFEATING PREMENSTRUAL SYNDROME (PMS) WITH EXPERT GUIDANCE

Ultimate Solution Handbook For Patients, Guardians Or Family To Understand, Manage, Treat, Prevent, Reverse Symptoms And Live Well

DR. POTTER WHITLEY

Copyright © 2023 by Dr. Potter Whitley

DISCLAIMER

This book's contents are meant to be used solely for informative purposes. The information should not be used as a replacement for expert medical advice, diagnosis, or care.

The information contained in this book is accurate and reliable, having been verified by the author to the best of his ability. Nevertheless, the author disclaims all express and implied representations and warranties regarding the availability, correctness, appropriateness, completeness, and reliability of the material provided here. You bear full responsibility for any reliance you may have on such material.

For informational purposes, this book may make reference to or mention of certain people, things, websites, organizations, or other names. The author has no connection to, endorsement from, or recommendation for these organizations. The author's approval or validation is not implied by the inclusion of these references.

Any direct, indirect, incidental, special, or consequential damages resulting from using or not being able to use the material in this book are not covered by the author's liability policy. For medical advice and counsel particular to their circumstances, readers are advised to check with experienced healthcare specialists.

The content, materials, and information in this book are subject to change at any time without prior notice, at the author's discretion. The text may contain errors or omissions for which the author is not responsible.

By reading this book, you understand and accept the conditions of this disclaimer.

THE REASON BEHIND THIS BOOK

"Defeating Premenstrual Syndrome (PMS) With Expert Guidance" is a priceless tool that explores the complex facets of PMS and offers a thorough manual for comprehending, treating, and eventually conquering this sometimes misdiagnosed ailment. To give readers a contextual understanding of PMS, this book begins with a thorough examination of historical viewpoints on the disease. The discussion then moves smoothly into a thorough analysis of the scientific foundations, explaining hormone fluctuations, neurotransmitter dynamics, and the interaction between hereditary and environmental influences.

This book's strength is its dedication to providing knowledge to empower others. The intricate process of identifying PMS patterns is explained to readers, enabling a customized method of symptom diagnosis and severity evaluation. The tale gains credibility from the expert perspectives of medical professionals, psychologists, and nutritionists, guaranteeing a comprehensive understanding of PMS and its effects on mental and physical health.

The comprehensive approach to PMS management in this book is one of its best qualities. The author offers readers a wide range of tools to incorporate into their wellness routines, from food choices stressing hormonal balance and superfoods to mind-body practices like yoga and meditation. Comprehensive lifestyle modifications are examined, including physical activity, proper sleep hygiene, and stress reduction methods, providing a comprehensive foundation for controlling PMS symptoms.

This book examines drugs and supplements in detail to address the pharmacological side of PMS. It guides readers through the maze of over-the-counter remedies, prescription drugs, and herbal supplements, giving them the information they need to make wise choices regarding their health. Mental health is not undervalued; this book gives helpful coping mechanisms and insightful information about the emotional health of people with PMS, highlighting the significance of receiving competent mental health care when necessary.

This book skillfully walks readers through several phases of life as it progresses, addressing the particular difficulties associated with PMS during youth, pregnancy, and menopause. Throughout, there is a strong sense of empowerment—people can manage and overcome PMS with the correct information, coping mechanisms, and assistance. The book ends with a section on self-empowerment, where readers are urged to assemble their own PMS toolkit, develop a strong support network, and acknowledge their accomplishments as they move toward long-term wellness. This book is more than just a manual; it is a source of empowerment and knowledge for everyone trying to overcome the obstacles that come with premenstrual syndrome.

TABLE OF CONTENT

CHAPTER ONE

UNDERSTANDING PREMENSTRUAL SYNDROME (PMS)
An Overview of PMS

A complex and varied disorder that affects many people who menstruate is called premenstrual syndrome, or PMS. It describes a group of behavioral, emotional, and physical symptoms that usually appear in the two weeks leading up to menstruation during the luteal phase of the menstrual cycle. A person's quality of life can be greatly impacted by PMS, which can affect everyday activities, relationships, and employment. It is critical to acknowledge that PMS is a common occurrence and that both those who are impacted by it and those in their vicinity must grasp its subtleties.

The primary cause of PMS is the hormonal changes that take place during the menstrual cycle. The fluctuating levels of progesterone and estrogen contribute to the range of symptoms felt. Although the precise etiology of PMS is unknown, it is thought that hormonal fluctuations affect neurotransmitters in the brain, which causes a variety of symptoms related to the disease. It is significant to remember that not everyone who menstruates gets PMS, and there can be significant variation in the intensity of symptoms.

Historical Views:

Examining Premenstrual Syndrome from historical viewpoints offers important insights into how this phenomenon has been seen and comprehended across time. In the past, PMS hasn't always been accepted as a real medical illness. Early narratives frequently blamed the symptoms on the emotional instability or even moral deficiencies of women. Medical practitioners did not start studying PMS as a serious and legitimate health concern until the late 20th century.

With the evolution of cultural views towards women's health, so too did our comprehension of PMS. The medical community began carrying out thorough investigations to determine the psychological and biological elements causing the condition. This change in viewpoint resulted in the creation of diagnostic standards and a more sophisticated comprehension of PMS as a multifaceted interaction between hormones, genetics, and environmental variables.

Typical Signs and Differences:

There is a broad spectrum of physical and emotional symptoms associated with premenstrual syndrome. Headaches, weariness, bloating, and breast tenderness are typical physical symptoms. Anxiety, depression, mood swings, and impatience are examples of emotional symptoms. The severity and length of these symptoms can differ amongst individuals; minor pain is experienced by some, while more severe indications are seen by others.

There are differences in PMS symptoms between people as well as within the same person over distinct menstrual cycles. In certain months, the symptoms could be negligible or nonexistent, while in other cycles, they might be crippling. Comprehending these variances is essential to managing PMS well. Every person's experience is different since several factors might affect the type and intensity of symptoms, including age, lifestyle, and general health.

In conclusion, a thorough grasp of this common yet sometimes misdiagnosed illness can be gained by exploring the introduction, historical viewpoints, and typical symptoms of PMS. This information serves as the cornerstone for successful therapies and support systems designed to enhance the well-being of PMS sufferers.

CHAPTER TWO

THE MECHANISMS UNDERLYING PMS
Changes in Hormones During the Menstruation Cycle:

The complicated dance between estrogen and progesterone controls the various hormonal swings that occur in a woman's body during her menstrual cycle. These hormones are in charge of the physiological changes that women go through during this time and are essential in controlling the menstrual cycle.

Estrogen levels rise in the early stages of the menstrual cycle, thickening the uterine lining in anticipation of a possible pregnancy. Luteinizing hormone, or LH, surges as ovulation gets closer, causing the ovary to produce an egg. Progesterone then increases to help the uterine lining and get the body ready for pregnancy.

Premenstrual syndrome (PMS) is thought to be triggered by changes in these hormones, namely the sharp drop in progesterone and estrogen levels during the premenstrual phase. Hormonal imbalance can cause a wide range of physical and psychological symptoms, from mood swings and irritation to bloating and breast tenderness. It has been discovered by researchers that each person's brain susceptibility to these hormone fluctuations varies, which affects how severe and how PMS symptoms appear. Knowing the complex hormonal dance that occurs during the menstrual cycle lays the groundwork for understanding the physiological causes of PMS.

PMS and Neurotransmitters:

The function of neurotransmitters in the brain adds another level of complexity to the understanding of premenstrual syndrome beyond changes in hormone levels. Mood-regulating chemical serotonin is specifically linked to the mood disorders that accompany PMS. Anger, melancholy, and anxiety are brought on by a drop in serotonin levels that occurs when estrogen levels fall during the premenstrual phase. It is believed that this neurotransmitter imbalance plays a role in the emotional and psychological symptoms that a lot of women go through during PMS.

Furthermore, PMS is linked to gamma-aminobutyric acid (GABA), a neurotransmitter that has inhibitory effects on the brain. Variations in GABA levels can worsen symptoms like anxiety and mood swings and make people more sensitive to stress. The complicated interplay between neurotransmitter activity and hormone changes highlights the multiple nature of PMS, where a complex web of symptoms is produced by the convergence of both hormonal and neurological variables.

Environmental and Genetic Factors:

Premenstrual syndrome (PMS) is primarily caused by hormonal fluctuations and neurotransmitter imbalances, although hereditary and environmental factors may contribute to the onset and intensity of PMS. Studies indicate that certain women may have a genetic susceptibility to variations in hormone levels and imbalances in neurotransmitters, which could lead to PMS. Gaining knowledge about the genetic foundations of PMS can be quite beneficial in determining how each person's symptoms emerge and intensify differently.

In addition, environmental variables including stress, food, and way of life might affect when PMS symptoms appear and how severe they get. For instance, long-term stress may intensify the effects of neurotransmitter swings and worsen hormone imbalances, producing more noticeable symptoms. Alcohol and caffeine intake are two more dietary decisions that may have an impact on PMS symptoms. Through an analysis of the complex interactions between genetic predispositions and environmental circumstances, scientists hope to decipher the complex network of variables that contribute to the variable character of PMS and open the door to more individualized and successful treatments.

CHAPTER THREE

IDENTIFYING PMS SYMPTOMS
Monitoring Monthly Cycles:

Understanding and monitoring menstrual cycles is essential to overcoming premenstrual syndrome (PMS). The intricate interaction of hormone fluctuations that occurs during a woman's menstrual cycle can have a big impact on her physical and mental health. People who keep a thorough menstrual calendar might start to identify patterns and predict when PMS symptoms will manifest. The beginning and ending dates of the menstrual cycle, along with any concomitant symptoms or mood swings, are all recorded during this tracking procedure. Modern technology has made tracking menstrual cycles easier, with a plethora of tools and applications available to help women learn more about their cycles over time.

Comprehending the subtleties of the menstrual cycle enables individuals to identify the stages during which symptoms of PMS are most likely to appear. Through the identification of the precise days or weeks preceding menstruation, people can take preemptive measures to alleviate the symptoms of PMS. This educated approach promotes a proactive mindset in tackling the difficulties presented by PMS, in addition to aiding in the management of symptoms and giving one a sense of control over their body.

Recognizing Individual Triggers

A tailored strategy is required to defeat PMS, one that includes determining and comprehending personal triggers. Women's PMS symptoms can differ greatly in form and severity. As a result, identifying the particular triggers that intensify symptoms becomes essential to creating a successful treatment strategy. A wide range of factors, such as food preferences, lifestyle choices, stress levels, and heredity, might be considered personal triggers.

A thorough self-evaluation is necessary to investigate the connection between these triggers and the onset of PMS symptoms. Meticulously documenting daily activities, emotions, and food consumption, helps people make links between particular triggers and the onset of PMS symptoms. Certain meals or drinks may serve as triggers for some people, while stress or sleep deprivation may be the main causes for others. Once recognized, these triggers can be controlled or avoided, enabling people to take proactive steps to lessen the negative effects of PMS on their general health.

Levels of Severity and Effect on Day-to-Day Living:

Developing coping strategies and looking for the right solutions require an understanding of the severity levels of PMS and how it affects day-to-day functioning. From minor irritability to more severe expressions like worry and depression, PMS symptoms can vary widely. Evaluating the influence of symptoms on relationships, employment, and general quality of life are some of the areas of daily living that are considered when assessing the severity of symptoms.

Modest symptom sufferers may find alleviation with dietary adjustments, stress reduction strategies, and lifestyle adjustments. However, for individuals who are dealing with more serious symptoms, consulting a physician is necessary. To address the impact of PMS on mental and emotional well-being, mental health specialists and healthcare providers can give customized interventions, such as cognitive-behavioral therapy or medication. Understanding the different levels of severity enables people to adjust their strategies so that the tactics they use correspond to the severity of their symptoms. This, in turn, makes for more efficient and individualized PMS management.

CHAPTER FOUR

PROFESSIONAL VIEWS ON PMS
Views from Medical Professionals:

Medical practitioners are essential in diagnosing and treating premenstrual syndrome (PMS). From a physiological perspective, PMS is defined by a variety of emotional and physical symptoms that arise during the menstrual cycle's luteal phase.

Endocrinologists and gynecologists frequently work together to investigate how a woman's health is affected by hormonal changes during this time. To correct hormonal imbalances and lessen PMS symptoms, doctors usually prescribe hormonal contraceptives, such as birth control tablets.

Medical experts also stress the significance of customized treatment regimens. Since each woman's experience with PMS is unique, successful management requires a customized strategy.

Hormone therapy may provide pain relief for some people, while nonsteroidal anti-inflammatory medications (NSAIDs) may be beneficial for others. Maintaining open lines of contact with medical professionals and scheduling routine checkups are crucial for tracking the efficacy of treatment and making necessary adjustments.

Moreover, a crucial component of medical intervention is addressing lifestyle variables. Promoting consistent exercise, getting enough sleep, and practicing stress reduction strategies can all help to reduce PMS symptoms. Healthcare providers emphasize that patients must take an active role in their health, using a comprehensive strategy that includes both medical treatments and lifestyle changes.

Psychologists' Perspectives on PMS and Mental Health:

Psychologists focus on the mental health elements of premenstrual syndrome, which gives them a unique perspective in the discussion of the disorder. Anxiety, irritability, and mood swings are frequently linked to PMS and can have a serious negative effect on a woman's psychological health. Psychologists emphasize the connection between hormonal changes and emotional states, noting that PMS is cyclical and can exacerbate pre-existing mental health issues.

One effective method for treating the psychological components of PMS is cognitive-behavioral therapy or CBT. CBT gives people the tools to recognize and question harmful thought patterns, which helps women deal with the emotional upheaval that comes with PMS. Psychologists also stress how crucial it is to create a supportive social and interpersonal environment for people to manage emotional triggers and stressors during the premenstrual period.

Psychologists also acknowledge that PMS may affect a person's ability to operate normally and their quality of life. To increase emotional resilience and enhance general mental health, methods like mindfulness and relaxation are frequently advised. Psychologists contribute to a holistic approach that goes beyond symptom management to enhance long-term mental health by treating the psychological aspects of PMS.

Suggestions from Nutritionists:

Nutritionists provide insightful advice on dietary tactics that can reduce discomfort and improve general well-being during the premenstrual period. Nutrition plays a critical part in controlling PMS symptoms. It is sometimes advised to have a balanced diet high in lean proteins, healthy fats, and complex carbs to stabilize blood sugar levels and lessen the mood fluctuations that are frequently linked to PMS.

Nutritionists stress that managing PMS requires consuming specific nutrients like calcium, magnesium, and vitamin B6. It is well-recognized that these nutrients affect the balance of hormones and relieve symptoms like irritation and bloating. Dietary items such as leafy greens, dairy products, nuts, and seeds can provide a natural source of these very important nutrients.

Nutritionists also recommend limiting alcohol, caffeine, and processed sweets because these might worsen PMS symptoms. It is also emphasized that maintaining proper hydration is essential to managing PMS, as it reduces bloating and promotes healthy physical functions.

Apart from providing nutritional advice, dietitians frequently work with individuals to develop customized nutrition regimens. Comprehending the distinct nutritional requirements and inclinations of every individual facilitates the creation of enduring and efficacious dietary approaches to handle PMS symptoms. Nutritionists contribute to a comprehensive strategy that enables people to handle the problems of PMS through thoughtful and health-conscious choices by fusing dietary expertise with lifestyle adjustments.

CHAPTER FIVE

COMPREHENSIVE METHODS FOR HANDLING PMS
Including Mind-Body Techniques

The incorporation of mind-body techniques is frequently highlighted in holistic approaches to PMS management as a successful strategy for reducing symptoms and enhancing general well-being. Deep breathing exercises and other mind-body techniques have been demonstrated to have a good effect on emotional stability and hormonal balance in the premenstrual period.

The development of mindfulness by meditation is a crucial component in combining mind-body techniques. Frequent meditation can help women become more self-aware and less stressed and anxious during their menstrual cycle. By encouraging people to remain in the present, mindfulness techniques help people develop emotional balance and serenity.

Since stress is a known trigger for PMS symptoms, integrating mindfulness into everyday activities can greatly help with symptom management.

Deep breathing techniques are essential for mind-body connection in addition to meditation. Intentional and controlled breathing exercises have been associated with lower cortisol levels and better hormonal balance. In addition to lowering stress, deep breathing improves the body's oxygenation, which may lessen PMS-related physical symptoms including bloating and exhaustion.

Moreover, mind-body practices encompass lifestyle choices that support holistic well-being in addition to individual techniques. A healthy diet, enough sleep, and regular exercise all support the general efficacy of mind-body integration. Participating in physical activities such as yoga or tai chi promotes a mind-body connection in addition to physical advantages, which is consistent with the holistic approach to PMS management.

In summary, adopting a holistic approach that includes mindfulness, meditation, and lifestyle choices is necessary for integrating mind-body activities. People who cultivate a mind-body connection may find that their PMS symptoms lessen, which will help to create a more harmonic and balanced menstrual cycle.

Yoga and Meditation to Alleviate PMS

When it comes to holistic PMS management, yoga, and meditation are particularly effective methods since they provide relief from both psychological and physical problems. Gentle movements, stretching, and controlled breathing are the main focuses of yoga, which is effective in reducing menstruation discomfort and enhancing general well-being.

Asanas, or yoga poses, created especially for PMS help with common problems including cramps, bloating, and tense muscles. These soft motions improve blood flow, which encourages relaxation and lessens the intensity of bodily discomfort. Furthermore, yoga's meditative elements promote mental calmness, which aids in assisting people in managing the mood swings and emotional fluctuations linked to PMS.

Whether done alone or in conjunction with yoga, meditation strengthens the mind-body connection that is essential for PMS relief. Emotional resilience is fostered by mindful meditation, which enables people to notice thoughts and feelings without passing judgment. Frequent meditation has been associated with lower stress hormone levels, which helps to create a more stable hormonal state before menstruation.

Furthermore, the rapid symptom relief that yoga and meditation provide is only one aspect of their comprehensive nature. Over time, regular practice increases both mental and physical toughness, which may eventually lessen the frequency and severity of PMS symptoms. By incorporating these routines into daily life, people can take charge of their health and foster a more positive relationship with their menstrual cycles.

By addressing both the physical and emotional components of premenstrual symptoms, yoga, and meditation together provide a comprehensive and empowering method of treating PMS.

Acupuncture and Complementary Medicine

Alternative therapies like acupuncture provide potential options for people looking for all-encompassing ways to control their PMS symptoms. With its roots in ancient Chinese medicine, acupuncture stimulates the flow of qi in the body by inserting tiny needles into particular spots. This method has demonstrated effectiveness in reducing a range of PMS symptoms, such as bloating, mood swings, and pain.

One of the main reasons acupuncture works so well for PMS relief is because of how it affects hormone control. Acupuncture helps balance the body's internal systems by affecting the release of hormones and neurotransmitters, which may lessen hormonal swings that worsen PMS symptoms. Furthermore, acupuncture's holistic philosophy treats PMS by treating underlying imbalances as well as its symptoms by viewing the body as a connected system.

A comprehensive strategy for managing PMS includes complementary therapies like nutritional supplements and herbal medication in addition to acupuncture. Herbal medicines that are natural and non-invasive alternatives to conventional treatments, such as chaste berry and evening primrose oil, have been examined for their potential to alleviate PMS symptoms. Dietary changes, such as consuming more omega-3 fatty acids and vitamin B6, may also help to lessen symptoms.

Many people report notable improvements in their PMS symptoms with acupuncture and other therapies, generally with fewer side effects than pharmaceutical interventions. However, individual reactions to these treatments vary. By incorporating these all-encompassing techniques into a thorough wellness program, people are given the ability to actively manage their PMS and take care of their physical and energetic well-being.

In summary, by treating underlying imbalances and enhancing general well-being, acupuncture, and alternative therapies provide comprehensive methods for PMS management.

These techniques add to a customized and all-encompassing approach for people looking for integrative and natural ways to ease the symptoms of premenstrual syndrome.

[35]

CHAPTER SIX

PMS DIETARY TECHNIQUES
Diet and Hormonal Harmony:

An important factor in preserving hormonal balance is proper diet, which also has a big impact on how severe PMS symptoms are. Throughout the menstrual cycle, hormones like progesterone and estrogen fluctuate, which can lead to the emotional and physical changes that many women go through. Include a diet rich in nutrients and well-rounded to maintain hormonal balance.

Important nutrients like omega-3 fatty acids, which are present in walnuts, flaxseeds, and fatty fish, can help control hormonal activity and lessen PMS-related inflammation. Furthermore, getting enough vitamin B6 from foods like chicken, bananas, and chickpeas might help produce neurotransmitters like serotonin, which helps reduce the irritability and mood swings that are frequently linked to PMS.

In addition, a diet high in antioxidants—found in a variety of vibrant fruits and vegetables—can help prevent oxidative stress and support hormonal balance in general. Berries, citrus fruits, and dark leafy greens are great options to boost the body's defense against free radical damage. In addition to promoting hormonal balance, a balanced diet improves general health and may lessen the effects of PMS on day-to-day functioning.

Superfoods to Alleviate PMS:

Some superfoods are particularly notable for their ability to mitigate PMS symptoms and offer comfort to individuals who are uncomfortable throughout their menstrual cycle. Ginger is one such superfood; it has anti-inflammatory qualities that can help reduce period cramps. One all-natural and practical method of managing PMS pain is to add ginger to beverages or meals.

Moreover, consuming foods high in magnesium, such as whole grains, nuts, and leafy greens, has been associated with a decrease in PMS symptoms. Magnesium can help relieve tension and bloating and is essential for relaxing muscles. By incorporating these superfoods into the diet, PMS can be managed holistically in addition to addressing individual symptoms.

The chaste tree berry, another well-known superfood, has long been utilized to promote the health of female reproduction. By affecting the pituitary gland, this herb may help balance hormones and maybe alleviate PMS symptoms like mood swings and breast soreness. Superfoods have their uses, but it's important to speak with a doctor to make sure they suit a person's dietary requirements and general health.

Planning Meals to Manage PMS:

Making a carefully considered diet plan is essential to controlling PMS symptoms. Meal planning reduces premenstrual syndrome discomfort while enabling people to make sure they are getting the nutrients they need to promote hormonal balance.

Maintaining a balanced intake of proteins, lipids, and carbohydrates along with an emphasis on whole foods can help stabilize blood sugar levels, which may lessen irritability and mood swings.

Including complex carbs in meals, such as those found in whole grains, legumes, and vegetables, can help reduce cravings for sugary snacks, which can aggravate PMS symptoms, and give a constant supply of energy. Lean protein sources including fish, chicken, and lentils as well as plant-based options like tofu can enhance general health and muscular performance.

Additionally, as it can support multiple bodily functions and reduce bloating, hydration is essential during PMS. Drinking water, drinking herbal teas, and eating foods high in water content, such as watermelon, can help you keep your fluid balance in check. All things considered, a careful and comprehensive food plan can play a major role in managing PMS and fostering mental and physical health during the menstrual cycle.

CHAPTER SEVEN

LIFESTYLE ADJUSTMENTS FOR PMS
Exercise and Physical Activity:

Frequent physical activity and exercise are essential for controlling and reducing premenstrual syndrome (PMS) symptoms. It has been demonstrated that maintaining a regular fitness regimen can improve mood, lessen bloating, and ease menstruation cramps. Exercises that increase heart rate, like jogging, cycling, or brisk walking, cause the body's natural mood enhancers, endorphins, to be released. These can help balance out the mood swings and irritation that are frequently linked to PMS.

Additionally, adding strength training activities to your regimen can help with muscle tone and general well-being. Improved circulation, which is another advantage of physical activity, may help lower water retention and lessen bloating and discomfort. Finding an exercise program that works for each person's tastes and talents is crucial because long-term benefits depend on consistency.

Exercise has many physical advantages, but it can also have a favorable effect on sleep patterns, which is another important factor in controlling PMS symptoms. Developing a regular exercise regimen also helps control hormone changes, which may be a factor in PMS symptoms, in addition to improving the quality of sleep.

PMS and Sleep Hygiene:

A good night's sleep is essential for maintaining general health and well-being, and it becomes even more important while managing the problems associated with premenstrual syndrome (PMS). Developing good sleep hygiene habits is essential to reducing the intensity of PMS symptoms. Improved sleep quality can be greatly aided by establishing a regular sleep pattern, keeping a cozy sleeping environment, and avoiding stimulants like electronics and coffee right before bed.

PMS is frequently accompanied by sleep difficulties; many women have symptoms like sleeplessness or irregular sleep patterns. These difficulties can be lessened by developing a peaceful, quiet, and dark sleeping environment as well as a calming bedtime ritual. Before going to bed, engaging in activities like deep breathing exercises or meditation can help you relax even more and make it easier to fall asleep.

Keeping a regular sleep schedule can also have a favorable impact on hormone balance, which may lessen PMS-related mood swings and irritation. Because sleep is essential for the body's healing process, making proper sleep hygiene a priority can help manage the overall effects of PMS on day-to-day functioning.

Techniques for Stress Management:

Reducing the negative effects of premenstrual syndrome (PMS) on one's physical and mental health requires practicing effective stress management.

Persistent stress can make PMS symptoms worse, making people more irritable, anxious, and physically uncomfortable. Therefore, developing a more resilient and balanced response to the hormonal swings that occur during the menstrual cycle requires the adoption of stress management practices.

It has been demonstrated that mindfulness exercises, like yoga and meditation, are beneficial in lowering stress and enhancing emotional well-being. By encouraging people to stay in the present, these methods make it easier for people to deal with the difficulties caused by PMS. Furthermore, useful techniques for encouraging relaxation and lowering general stress levels are gradual muscle relaxation and deep breathing exercises.

Regular pauses and recreational activities incorporated into everyday schedules can also help reduce stress. Finding enjoyable and relaxing hobbies or pastimes, such as reading or spending time in nature, can have a favorable effect on one's general mental health.

Developing a network of social contacts and honest communication can act as an emotional support system during trying times and help people feel resilient when faced with stressors connected to PMS.

[47]

CHAPTER EIGHT

PMS SUPPLEMENTS AND MEDICATIONS
Over-the-Counter PMS Medications:

Premenstrual syndrome (PMS) sufferers can find easily available and easy treatment for the symptoms of the condition with over-the-counter (OTC) solutions. Nonsteroidal anti-inflammatory drugs (NSAIDs), such as ibuprofen and naproxen, are nonprescription pharmaceuticals that are frequently used to treat PMS-related pain, such as headaches and menstrual cramps. These drugs provide women with menstrual period discomfort with significant relief by decreasing inflammation and inhibiting pain signals.

To treat symptoms like bloating and breast discomfort, antihistamines like diphenhydramine can be used in addition to NSAIDs. These drugs assist in controlling water retention and reduce some of the pain associated with menstrual irregularities.

Moreover, diuretics—which are sold over-the-counter—may help lessen bloating by encouraging the elimination of extra fluid. For women looking for non-prescription treatment for certain PMS symptoms, these over-the-counter solutions offer a variety of possibilities.

Although many people find success with over-the-counter (OTC) choices, it is important to speak with a healthcare provider before using them, particularly if there are any pre-existing medical conditions or concerns about possible drug interactions. To prevent side effects, it's also crucial to closely adhere to dosing directions.

Medication prescribed for PMS:

Prescription drugs may provide more focused and effective relief for people with severe or ongoing PMS symptoms. Selective serotonin reuptake inhibitors are one class of medications that are frequently administered (SSRIs). It has been discovered that these antidepressants, which include sertraline and fluoxetine, reduce mood-related PMS symptoms by raising serotonin levels in the brain. This may lessen the anger, anxiety, and depression that PMS is known to cause.

Another prescription option is gonadotropin-releasing hormone agonists or GnRH agonists. These drugs perform by inhibiting ovarian function and momentarily causing menopause. Even while this method is not recommended for long-term use, it can significantly help ladies who are experiencing severe PMS symptoms.

Hormonal contraceptives, like birth control pills, may be administered in some situations to moderate changes in hormone levels and lessen PMS symptoms. By stabilizing estrogen and progesterone levels, these contraceptives can lessen mood swings, bloating, and other related discomforts.

Those who are thinking about using prescription drugs for PMS should speak with their healthcare professional in-depth. To choose the best course of action, potential advantages and disadvantages as well as specific health factors should be thoroughly considered.

Vitamins and Herbal Supplements for PMS:

The use of vitamins and herbal supplements as a natural way to treat PMS symptoms has gained popularity in recent years. Numerous dietary supplements have demonstrated the potential to offer alleviation without the negative effects linked to traditional pharmaceuticals.

The fruit of the chaste tree is the source of chasteberry, a well-liked herbal treatment. It is thought that chaste berry influences hormone levels, specifically the ratio of progesterone to estrogen. According to studies, chasteberry may lessen PMS symptoms like headaches, mood swings, and breast soreness.

Another supplement that has drawn interest for its possible function in managing PMS is magnesium, a mineral that is involved in many physiological processes.

According to certain research, taking a magnesium supplement may help with PMS-related bloating, breast pain, and mood swings.

Studies have also looked into the possibility of vitamin B6, which is present in foods like fish, poultry, and bananas, reducing the symptoms of PMS. Because this vitamin is involved in the synthesis of neurotransmitters, taking supplements may help control mood and lessen symptoms like depression and irritability.

Although vitamins and herbal supplements provide a more natural solution, it's important to use caution when using them. It is advisable to speak with a healthcare provider about dosages and possible drug interactions. Furthermore, each person may react differently to these supplements, and their effectiveness may not always be the same.

In conclusion, a thorough strategy for treating PMS symptoms involves investigating over-the-counter products, prescription drugs, herbal supplements, and vitamins.

To find the best and most efficient combination of treatments for their unique requirements and medical problems, people must collaborate closely with healthcare specialists.

CHAPTER NINE

MENTAL HEALTH AND PMS
PMS and Emotional Wellness

The menstrual cycle and emotional well-being are closely related, and the premenstrual period can pose serious difficulties for many women. Emotional symptoms, which can vary from mood swings and irritation to anxiety and depression, are a common manifestation of premenstrual syndrome (PMS). Comprehending and regulating emotional welfare throughout this stage is essential for general psychological well-being.

Changes in mood and emotional states can result from the premenstrual hormone changes' significant effects on neurotransmitters in the brain. Rises and falls in estrogen and progesterone levels affect serotonin, a neurotransmitter linked to mood control. Because of the potential for these hormonal shifts to intensify emotional reactions, people must pay close attention to their mental health throughout this period.

Developing self-awareness is essential to preserving emotional stability during PMS. Identifying triggers and tracking emotional patterns in a notebook can yield insightful information. Deep breathing, meditation, and yoga are examples of relaxation techniques that can help reduce stress and emotional problems. Emotional stability can also be facilitated by leading a balanced lifestyle that includes frequent exercise and nutritious food.

Creating a network of support is essential for maintaining emotional health during PMS. Understanding and empathy can be fostered by being open and honest about the difficulties encountered in this era with friends, family, or partners. By providing a secure environment for people to express their feelings, emotional symptoms might be lessened.

In conclusion, managing stress, developing a supporting network, and self-awareness are all important components of treating emotional well-being during PMS. Through proactive measures to comprehend and handle emotional symptoms, people can more easily traverse the premenstrual phase, thus enhancing their general mental health and well-being.

Coping Mechanisms for Symptoms of Emotion

Managing the affective symptoms linked to PMS necessitates a multifaceted strategy that enables people to successfully negotiate the obstacles. Although each person's emotional symptoms may present differently, there are common tactics that can be used to lessen the impact and improve coping mechanisms.

First and foremost, it's critical to create a regimen that includes stress-relieving activities. Exercise regularly has been demonstrated to improve mood and reduce emotional symptoms. Emotional relief can be obtained by indulging in enjoyable and soothing activities like reading, listening to music, or going outside.

Cognitive-behavioral methods and mindfulness are useful coping mechanisms for emotional problems. Deep breathing exercises and meditation are examples of mindfulness activities that assist people in managing their emotions and remaining in the present moment. To promote emotional resilience, cognitive-behavioral techniques entail recognizing negative thought patterns and swapping them out for more productive and positive ones.

During PMS, emotional symptoms can be effectively managed by dietary choices. Mood can be improved by eating a diet rich in complex carbs, lean proteins, and enough vitamins and minerals. It's critical to limit alcohol, sugar, and caffeine intake as these chemicals can aggravate emotional symptoms.

It's critical to recognize the value of self-compassion in this trying time. It is empowering to acknowledge that emotional symptoms are a normal aspect of the menstrual cycle rather than a sign of weakness. A feeling of solidarity and validation can be obtained by reaching out for social support and making connections with people who might be going through comparable struggles.

In conclusion, a comprehensive strategy that incorporates lifestyle modifications, mindfulness exercises, and self-compassion is needed to manage the emotional symptoms of PMS. Through the integration of these tactics into their everyday routines, people can proficiently handle emotional obstacles, cultivating a more optimistic and robust perspective.

Getting Help for Mental Health Professionals

Although self-help techniques might be helpful, there are situations in which getting professional mental health treatment is essential for handling PMS-related difficulties. Professional assistance can provide people with the skills and coping strategies they need to manage their emotional symptoms and enhance their general mental health.

Getting help through psychotherapy is one option. The emotional symptoms of PMS can be effectively treated with cognitive-behavioral therapy (CBT). CBT assists people in recognizing and altering harmful thought patterns, creating constructive coping mechanisms, and improving emotional control. Therapy solutions can be specifically designed by a qualified mental health practitioner to address the unique requirements and difficulties encountered during the premenstrual period.

A mental health practitioner may occasionally advise medication to treat severe emotional issues. Mood stabilizers and antidepressants can help control neurotransmitters and lessen the negative effects of hormone changes on mood. It's crucial to speak with a healthcare professional about the advantages and disadvantages of taking medicine depending on your unique situation.

Support groups can be a great resource as well. Developing ties with people who have gone through comparable things fosters understanding and a sense of community. A more all-encompassing and encouraging approach to treating PMS-related emotional problems can involve exchanging coping mechanisms, showing empathy, and taking inspiration from the experiences of others.

In conclusion, people who are experiencing serious problems related to PMS should take the proactive measure of obtaining professional mental health support. By providing expert advice, whether through psychotherapy, medication, or support group involvement, emotional symptoms can be better managed, leading to a more robust and self-assured approach to mental health.

[61]

CHAPTER TEN

NAVIGATING PMS IN DIFFERENT LIFE STAGES
PMS in Adolescence

A woman's adolescence is a crucial time in her life, characterized by changes in her body and hormones. Premenstrual syndrome (PMS) often begins during this phase for many young girls, which adds another level of difficulty to an already difficult time. Adolescent PMS can present with a range of symptoms, including mood swings, irritability, and somatic complaints such as breast soreness and bloating. Teenagers may experience more noticeable hormonal variations during their menstrual cycle, which can exacerbate PMS symptoms.

Managing PMS during adolescence calls for a sophisticated strategy. PMS symptoms are largely a result of hormonal changes, and educating young girls about these changes might help them get through this transitional stage more easily. Adolescents can feel more supported and less alone in their experiences if parents, educators, and medical professionals are encouraged to have open conversations regarding PMS.

Furthermore, dietary habits, physical activity, and stress reduction can have a big impact on how severe PMS symptoms are in teenagers. Educating teenagers on the value of self-care routines and a healthy lifestyle can enable them to actively manage their PMS. Additionally, getting expert advice from a gynecologist or mental health specialist can offer customized coping mechanisms for the particular difficulties associated with PMS in adolescence.

Pregnancy and PMS

Many women find pregnancy to be a miraculous and life-changing experience, but it also brings with it a unique set of hormonal changes that may interact with symptoms of premenstrual syndrome (PMS). Pregnancy might cause some women's PMS symptoms to lessen, while it can also cause some women to become more sensitive. Pregnancy and PMS have a complicated relationship that differs from woman to woman.

To effectively manage PMS symptoms, one must comprehend the interaction between normal menstrual cycle and hormonal changes during pregnancy. Changes in hormones, especially the increase in progesterone during pregnancy, can affect mood, vitality, and physical health. This hormone change may provide some women a much-needed break from the typical PMS symptoms during pregnancy. Others, though, might discover that the distinct hormonal environment of pregnancy presents a different set of difficulties.

Pregnancy-related PMS management calls for customized care. It is crucial to speak with a healthcare provider to determine the exact situation and suggest the best course of action for managing symptoms. A more joyful pregnancy experience can also be achieved by taking a holistic approach that incorporates a healthy lifestyle, enough nourishment, and emotional support—even in the event of PMS symptoms.

PMS and Menopause

A woman's journey through menopause, the biological process that naturally signals the end of her menstrual cycle, is marked by an important turning point. Although PMS is usually linked to the reproductive years, some women may still have symptoms similar to PMS during perimenopause, which is the period of transition before menopause. PMS-like symptoms might arise from hormonal imbalances and fluctuations that are specific to perimenopause, which can mimic the hormonal changes that occur throughout the menstrual cycle.

Managing PMS throughout the perimenopause necessitates a thorough comprehension of the particular difficulties this stage of life presents. Under the supervision of a medical expert, hormone replacement therapy (HRT) may be investigated as a means of reducing symptoms related to PMS and perimenopause.

During this period of transition, lifestyle improvements such as consistent exercise, a well-balanced diet, and effective stress management are essential for maintaining overall well-being.

Furthermore, it is impossible to ignore the psychological effects of PMS and the perimenopause. Women can be empowered to overcome obstacles with grace and resilience by receiving emotional support, therapy, and information about the physiological changes that are taking place during this time. Understanding that menopause signifies not just the end of reproductive potential but also a significant change in general health and well-being guarantees a comprehensive strategy for treating PMS symptoms throughout this phase of life.

CHAPTER ELEVEN

TAKING CHARGE OF YOUR RECOVERY FROM PMS
Building a Customized PMS Toolbox

Premenstrual syndrome (PMS) can be defeated in part by creating a customized toolbox that addresses each person's unique needs and symptoms. This toolkit is an all-inclusive resource for managing PMS-related physical and mental difficulties. Begin by pinpointing particular symptoms that affect your day-to-day functioning, such as mood swings, anger, exhaustion, or physical discomfort.

To address emotional well-being, think about adding stress-relieving methods to your repertoire, such as yoga, meditation, or deep breathing exercises. Modifying one's diet to include cutting back on sugar and caffeine can also have a big impact on how well PMS symptoms are managed.

Investigate complementary therapies like herbal supplements or acupuncture in addition to traditional therapies. Maintain a notebook to monitor your symptoms and spot trends and triggers. This will help you manage your PMS proactively rather than reactively. With time, your toolbox should adjust to your changing lifestyle and symptoms. To guarantee its efficacy, review and update it frequently. You can equip yourself with a customized set of techniques to deal with the difficulties that come up during the various stages of your menstrual cycle by making a unique PMS toolbox.

Establishing a Network of Support

Having a strong support network is essential to overcoming PMS because it offers emotional, practical, and informational support when things get hard. To promote understanding and empathy, be transparent about your PMS experience with friends, family, and coworkers. Dispel myths and misconceptions about PMS to enable your support network to offer knowledgeable and empathetic assistance.

Promote candid conversations about your unique requirements during PMS, including extra help with chores, a sympathetic ear, or just a little space when needed. Having a support system of people who value and comprehend your experience can go a long way toward reducing the emotional toll that PMS takes. Seek expert advice from medical professionals, therapists, or women's health-focused support groups to acquire more understanding and coping skills.

Integrate your support network into your day-to-day activities to foster a sense of belonging and shared accountability. A solid support network is essential for overcoming the difficulties associated with PMS, whether that support takes the form of going to social gatherings with others, participating in stress-relieving activities, or just having someone to ask how you're doing. You give yourself an invaluable tool that enhances your general well-being by actively creating and maintaining this support system.

Honoring Development and Prolonged Well-Being

It takes time to overcome PMS, and acknowledging your accomplishments is essential to keeping your motivation high and preserving your progress. Celebrate little successes, such as putting a new coping strategy into practice or seeing a decrease in the intensity of symptoms. By concentrating on your successes, you strengthen your capacity to actively handle and go past the obstacles posed by PMS.

For your road towards PMS management, think about establishing reasonable and doable objectives. This could include adopting regular exercise, adhering to a constant self-care regimen, or gradually changing one's nutrition. Celebrate your progress and accomplishments to reaffirm your dedication to long-term wellness. Recognize that beating PMS is a dynamic process needing constant work and adaptability. Evaluate your progress regularly and revise your goals as necessary.

Include positive reinforcement in your self-care regimen. For example, give yourself a treat when you maintain a healthy habit or consult a professional when necessary. By acknowledging your accomplishments and making a commitment to long-term fitness, you give yourself the strength to overcome PMS obstacles and maintain an optimistic outlook. Recall that managing PMS is a non-linear process and that you can cultivate a sense of empowerment and control over your health by praising yourself for your accomplishments.